NO GALLBLADDER COOKBOOK FOR SENIORS

Tasty and Easy Recipes to Restore Your Health

MEY W SMITH

TABLE

Introduction

The "No Gallbladder Cookbook for Seniors" addresses the dietary challenges faced by individuals who have undergone gallbladder removal surgery, a common procedure among seniors. This cookbook aims to provide practical and nutritious recipes tailored to support digestive health in the absence of the gallbladder. Understanding the types of recipes, the causes leading to gallbladder removal, associated symptoms, and preventive measures are crucial components in comprehending the significance of such a cookbook for seniors.

Types of Recipes

The cookbook typically includes recipes that focus on low-fat and easily digestible foods. Since the gallbladder is responsible for storing and releasing bile to aid in fat digestion, individuals without a gallbladder may experience difficulties digesting large amounts of fat. Therefore, recipes in the cookbook emphasize lean proteins, vegetables, and complex carbohydrates. Additionally, the cookbook might feature meals that incorporate digestive-friendly herbs and spices to enhance flavor without compromising health.

Causes of Gallbladder Removal

Gallbladder removal, or cholecystectomy, is often necessitated by conditions such as gallstones, inflammation, or infection. Gallstones, formed when substances in bile harden, can obstruct the flow of bile and cause pain. Inflammation of the gallbladder, known as cholecystitis, can result from gallstones or other factors. In some cases, infection or dysfunction may prompt the need for gallbladder removal. Understanding these causes is essential for seniors and their caregivers to manage post-surgery dietary needs effectively.

Symptoms After Gallbladder Removal

Post-cholecystectomy, individuals may experience changes in digestion. Common symptoms include diarrhea, bloating, and discomfort after consuming fatty foods. The absence of a gallbladder affects the regulation of bile, impacting the efficient breakdown of fats. The cookbook addresses these symptoms by providing recipes that promote easy digestion and minimize the risk of triggering discomfort.

Preventive Measures

Preventive measures for seniors without a gallbladder revolve around dietary adjustments. These can include eating smaller, more frequent meals to reduce the load on the digestive system, emphasizing soluble fiber intake to regulate bowel movements, and avoiding high-fat foods. The cookbook serves as a guide, offering recipes designed to adhere to these preventive measures and support overall digestive well-being.

The "No Gallbladder Cookbook for Seniors" plays a crucial role in assisting individuals who have undergone gallbladder removal surgery. By focusing on types of recipes that align with post-surgery dietary needs, addressing the causes leading to gallbladder removal, understanding symptoms associated with its absence, and providing preventive measures, the cookbook serves as a valuable resource for seniors seeking to maintain a healthy and satisfying diet despite the challenges posed by gallbladder removal.

Chapter 1

What to eat or not

The "No Gallbladder Cookbook for Seniors" emphasizes specific foods to include and avoid, catering to the unique dietary needs of individuals who have undergone gallbladder removal surgery. This cookbook aims to support digestive health by recommending foods that are easily digestible and minimizing those that may trigger discomfort. Here's a breakdown of the key considerations for food choices in the cookbook:

Foods to Include

1. -Lean Proteins- Seniors without a gallbladder are encouraged to include lean protein sources in their diet. These may include poultry, fish, tofu, and legumes. Lean proteins help maintain muscle mass and provide essential nutrients without overloading the digestive system with excessive fats.

2. -Low-Fat Dairy- The cookbook suggests incorporating low-fat or fat-free dairy products to meet calcium and vitamin D needs. Examples include skim milk, yogurt, and reduced-fat cheese. These options provide essential nutrients without the high-fat content that may be challenging to digest.

3. -Fruits and Vegetables- A variety of fruits and vegetables are recommended, as they offer fiber and essential vitamins. However, attention is given to choosing those that are low in fat and easy to digest. Bananas, apples, carrots, and leafy greens are examples of digestive-friendly options.

4. -Whole Grains- The cookbook promotes the inclusion of whole grains, such as brown rice, quinoa, and oats. These grains provide fiber for digestive health while being lower in fat compared to refined grains. Fiber aids in regulating bowel movements and supporting overall gut function.

5. -Healthy Fats- While a gallbladder is no longer present to assist in fat digestion, incorporating small amounts of healthy fats is still recommended. Olive oil, avocados, and nuts can be included in moderation. These sources of fats are easier on the digestive system compared to saturated and trans fats.

Foods to Avoid

1. -High-Fat Foods- The cookbook advises seniors to steer clear of high-fat foods, as these can lead to digestive discomfort. Fried foods, fatty cuts of meat, and rich desserts should be minimized or avoided to prevent overloading the digestive system with fats that are challenging to process.

2. -Processed Foods- Highly processed and refined foods often contain hidden fats, additives, and preservatives.

Seniors are encouraged to choose whole, minimally processed options to promote better digestion and overall health.

3. -Spicy Foods- Spices and spicy foods may trigger digestive issues in individuals without a gallbladder. The cookbook suggests limiting the use of strong spices and opting for milder alternatives to enhance flavor without causing discomfort.

4. -Excessive Caffeine and Alcohol- Seniors are advised to moderate their intake of caffeine and alcohol, as these substances can irritate the digestive tract. The cookbook encourages choosing decaffeinated options and limiting alcohol consumption to support digestive well-being.

5. -Large Meals- Consuming large meals can overwhelm the digestive system, leading to discomfort. The cookbook recommends seniors opt for smaller, more frequent meals to support efficient digestion and minimize the risk of digestive issues.

In essence, the "No Gallbladder Cookbook for Seniors" provides practical guidance on food choices that align with the unique dietary needs of individuals who have undergone gallbladder removal surgery

Benefits

Following a diet tailored for individuals without a gallbladder, as outlined in the "No Gallbladder Cookbook for Seniors," offers several core benefits aimed at supporting digestive health and overall well-being. Here are key advantages:

1. -Digestive Comfort-
   - Explanation- The absence of a gallbladder can lead to challenges in digesting fats effectively. The cookbook focuses on recipes that are lower in fat and easier on the digestive system, reducing the likelihood of discomfort, bloating, and other digestive issues commonly experienced after gallbladder removal.

2. -Nutrient Absorption-
   - Explanation- The cookbook emphasizes nutrient-dense foods, ensuring seniors receive essential vitamins and minerals despite the altered digestive environment. By including a variety of fruits, vegetables, lean proteins, and whole grains, the diet supports optimal nutrient absorption, addressing potential deficiencies that may arise after gallbladder surgery.

3. -Balanced Nutrition-
   - Explanation- Maintaining a balanced diet is crucial for overall health, especially for seniors. The cookbook provides a variety of recipes that include the necessary components of

a well-rounded diet, such as proteins, carbohydrates, fats (in moderation), vitamins, and minerals. This balanced approach supports seniors in meeting their nutritional requirements.

4. -Stable Blood Sugar Levels-
   - Explanation- The cookbook recommends incorporating complex carbohydrates and avoiding highly processed foods, contributing to stable blood sugar levels. This is particularly beneficial for seniors, as it helps prevent energy crashes and supports overall energy management throughout the day.

5. -Weight Management-
   - Explanation- The focus on lean proteins, whole grains, and a reduction in high-fat foods can aid in weight management for seniors. Maintaining a healthy weight is essential for various aspects of well-being, including cardiovascular health, joint function, and overall mobility.

6. -Improved Bowel Regularity-
   - Explanation- Including fiber-rich foods from fruits, vegetables, and whole grains helps regulate bowel movements. Seniors without a gallbladder may experience changes in digestion, and the cookbook's emphasis on fiber contributes to improved bowel regularity and digestive comfort.

7. -Heart Health Support-

- Explanation- The inclusion of heart-healthy fats, such as those found in olive oil, avocados, and nuts, supports cardiovascular health. Seniors often face increased risks related to heart health, and the cookbook's recommendations align with a heart-healthy diet, contributing to overall well-being.

8. -Reduced Risk of Gallstone Formation-

- Explanation- The cookbook's emphasis on a low-fat diet reduces the risk of gallstone formation post-gallbladder removal. By avoiding excessive dietary fats, seniors can minimize the likelihood of complications related to gallstones, promoting long-term digestive health.

9. -Enhanced Flavor Without Discomfort-

- Explanation- The cookbook incorporates herbs and spices that enhance flavor without causing digestive discomfort. This allows seniors to enjoy their meals without compromising on taste, creating a positive and satisfying culinary experience.

10. -Support for Aging Gracefully-

- Explanation- As individuals age, dietary considerations become increasingly important for maintaining health and vitality. The "No Gallbladder Cookbook for Seniors" provides practical solutions tailored to the specific needs of seniors who have undergone gallbladder removal, supporting them in aging gracefully with a focus on digestive wellness.

the "No Gallbladder Cookbook for Seniors" offers a range of core benefits, including improved digestive comfort, balanced nutrition, stable blood sugar levels, weight management, heart health support, and reduced risk of gallstone formation. These advantages contribute to an overall positive impact on the well-being of seniors navigating life without a gallbladder.

Chapter 2

Shopping ingredients

1. -Lean Proteins-
   - Explanation- Include skinless poultry, fish, lean cuts of meat, and plant-based protein sources like tofu and legumes. These provide essential nutrients without excessive fat content, supporting seniors in maintaining muscle mass and overall health.

2. -Low-Fat Dairy-
   - Explanation- Opt for low-fat or fat-free dairy products such as skim milk, yogurt, and reduced-fat cheese. These choices offer necessary calcium and vitamin D without the added burden of high-fat content.

3. -Fruits-
   - Explanation- Choose a variety of fruits, including bananas, apples, berries, and melons. These fruits are not only rich in vitamins and antioxidants but also tend to be lower in fat and gentle on the digestive system.

4. -Vegetables-
   - Explanation- Prioritize a colorful array of vegetables, such as leafy greens, carrots, broccoli, and bell peppers.

Vegetables contribute essential fiber, vitamins, and minerals while being low in fat and easily digestible.

5. -Whole Grains-

   - Explanation- Include whole grains like brown rice, quinoa, oats, and whole wheat bread. These grains offer fiber, aiding in digestion and providing sustained energy without the excess fat found in refined grains.

6. -Healthy Fats-

   - Explanation- Choose sources of healthy fats like olive oil, avocados, and nuts. These fats are easier on the digestive system and provide essential fatty acids without overloading the body with saturated or trans fats.

7. -Herbs and Spices-

   - Explanation- Incorporate digestive-friendly herbs and spices like ginger, mint, turmeric, and parsley. These not only add flavor to meals but may also have anti-inflammatory properties, supporting digestive health.

8. -Eggs-

   - Explanation- Include eggs as a versatile protein source. Eggs are generally well-tolerated and can be prepared in various ways, providing seniors with a nutrient-dense option for meals.

9. -Low-Fat Condiments-

- Explanation- Choose low-fat or fat-free condiments such as mustard, salsa, and vinegar-based dressings. These add flavor to meals without contributing to excessive fat intake.

10. -Greek Yogurt-
   - Explanation- Opt for Greek yogurt, which is rich in protein and probiotics. Probiotics can be beneficial for gut health, aiding digestion and supporting a balanced microbiome.

11. -Whole Wheat Pasta-
   - Explanation- Select whole wheat pasta as a fiber-rich alternative to traditional pasta. This supports digestive health and provides a heartier option for meals.

12. -Lean Cuts of Meat-
   - Explanation- Choose lean cuts of meat, such as skinless poultry or lean beef. Trimming visible fat before cooking reduces the overall fat content, making these proteins more easily digestible.

13. -Sweet Potatoes-
   - Explanation- Incorporate sweet potatoes as a nutrient-dense, low-fat source of carbohydrates. They are rich in vitamins and fiber, promoting digestive health.

14. -Salmon-

- Explanation- Include fatty fish like salmon, which provides omega-3 fatty acids. These healthy fats support heart health and may have anti-inflammatory effects.

15. -Chia Seeds-
-Explanation- Add chia seeds to meals or snacks for a boost of omega-3 fatty acids, fiber, and protein. Chia seeds can be sprinkled on yogurt, added to smoothies, or used in baking.

16. -Lentils-
-Explanation- Incorporate lentils into soups, stews, or salads. They are a rich source of plant-based protein and fiber, contributing to digestive well-being.

17. -Low-Sodium Broth-
-Explanation- Use low-sodium broth as a base for soups and stews. It adds flavor without excessive salt, promoting heart health and overall well-being.

18. -Cauliflower Rice-
-Explanation- Opt for cauliflower rice as a low-carb alternative to traditional rice. It's a versatile option that can be used in various dishes while being lower in fat.

19. -Berries-
-Explanation- Enjoy a variety of berries like blueberries, strawberries, and raspberries. Berries are rich in antioxidants and low in fat, making them a nutritious and flavorful addition to meals or snacks.

20. -Green Tea-
 -Explanation- Choose green tea for a hydrating, low-calorie beverage. Green tea is rich in antioxidants and has potential health benefits, supporting seniors in maintaining overall well-being.

these 20 healthy shopping ingredients for a "No Gallbladder Cookbook for Seniors" are selected to provide a well-rounded, nutrient-dense, and easily digestible diet. Incorporating these ingredients into meals supports seniors in managing their digestive health and overall nutritional needs post-gallbladder removal.

BREAKFAST

1. Protein-Packed Scrambled Eggs with Spinach

-Ingredients-
- 2 eggs
- 1 cup fresh spinach, chopped
- Salt and pepper to taste

-Preparation-
- Whisk eggs and fold in chopped spinach.
- Cook on a non-stick pan over medium heat until eggs are cooked through.

-Nutritional Value-
- Protein: 12g
- Calories: 180
- Cooking Time: 5 minutes

2. Greek Yogurt Parfait with Berries

-Ingredients-
- 1 cup Greek yogurt
- 1/2 cup mixed berries (blueberries, strawberries)
- 2 tablespoons granola

-Preparation-
- Layer Greek yogurt, berries, and granola in a glass.
- Repeat for a delightful parfait.

-Nutritional Value-
- Protein: 15g
- Fiber: 4g
- Calories: 250
- Cooking Time: 2 minutes

3. Oatmeal with Almond Butter and Banana

-Ingredients-
- 1/2 cup rolled oats
- 1 cup water or milk
- 1 tablespoon almond butter
- 1/2 banana, sliced

-Preparation-
- Cook oats with water or milk until desired consistency.
- Top with almond butter and banana slices.

-Nutritional Value-
- Fiber: 5g
- Protein: 8g
- Calories: 280
- Cooking Time: 7 minutes

4. Whole Wheat Avocado Toast with Poached Egg

-Ingredients-
- 1 slice whole wheat bread
- 1/2 avocado, mashed
- 1 egg (poached)
- Salt and pepper to taste

-Preparation-
- Toast bread, spread mashed avocado, and top with a poached egg.

-Nutritional Value-
- Protein: 10g
- Fiber: 6g
- Calories: 280
- Cooking Time: 10 minutes

5. Cottage Cheese and Pineapple Bowl

-Ingredients-
- 1/2 cup low-fat cottage cheese
- 1/2 cup fresh pineapple, diced
- 1 tablespoon honey

-Preparation-
- Combine cottage cheese and pineapple in a bowl.
- Drizzle with honey.

-Nutritional Value-
    - Protein: 15g
    - Vitamin C: 40mg
    - Calories: 200
    - Preparation Time: 5 minutes

6. Smoothie Bowl with Spinach and Berry Blend

-Ingredients-
    - 1 cup spinach
    - 1/2 cup mixed berries (strawberries, blueberries)
    - 1/2 cup Greek yogurt
    - 1/2 cup almond milk

-Preparation-
    - Blend spinach, berries, yogurt, and almond milk until smooth.
    - Pour into a bowl and add desired toppings.

-Nutritional Value-
    - Protein: 12g
    - Fiber: 6g
    - Calories: 220
    - Preparation Time: 5 minutes

7. Quinoa Breakfast Bowl with Almond Milk

-Ingredients-

- 1/2 cup cooked quinoa
- 1/4 cup almonds, sliced
- 1/2 cup almond milk
- 1 tablespoon honey

-Preparation-
- Combine cooked quinoa, sliced almonds, almond milk, and drizzle with honey.

-Nutritional Value-
- Protein: 8g
- Fiber: 5g
- Calories: 280
- Cooking Time: 15 minutes (including quinoa prep)

8. Chia Seed Pudding with Mango

-Ingredients-
- 2 tablespoons chia seeds
- 1/2 cup almond milk
- 1/2 mango, diced

-Preparation-
- Mix chia seeds and almond milk, let sit overnight.
- Top with diced mango before serving.

-Nutritional Value-
- Fiber: 10g

- Protein: 6g
- Calories: 220
- Preparation Time: 5 minutes (plus overnight soak)

9. Turkey and Veggie Breakfast Wrap

-Ingredients-
- 1 whole wheat tortilla
- 2 slices turkey breast
- 1 egg (scrambled)
- 1/4 cup bell peppers, diced

-Preparation-
- Cook scrambled eggs and bell peppers, assemble in a tortilla with turkey.

-Nutritional Value-
- Protein: 15g
- Fiber: 4g
- Calories: 280
- Cooking Time: 8 minutes

10. Sweet Potato and Apple Hash

-Ingredients-
- 1 sweet potato, grated
- 1 apple, diced
- 1 tablespoon olive oil
- Cinnamon to taste

-Preparation-
- Sauté grated sweet potato and diced apple in olive oil until cooked.
- Sprinkle with cinnamon before serving.

-Nutritional Value-
- Fiber: 6g
- Vitamin A: 250% DV
- Calories: 220
- Cooking Time: 10 minutes

These breakfast recipes from the "No Gallbladder Cookbook for Seniors" are designed to provide a balance of nutrients, support digestive health, and offer delicious options for seniors following a gallbladder-friendly diet. Adjust portion sizes based on individual nutritional needs

LUNCH

1. Grilled Lemon Herb Chicken Breast

-Ingredients-
- 4 boneless, skinless chicken breasts
- 2 tablespoons olive oil
- 1 lemon (juiced)
- 1 teaspoon dried oregano
- 1 teaspoon dried thyme
- Salt and pepper to taste

-Preparation-
1. In a bowl, mix olive oil, lemon juice, oregano, thyme, salt, and pepper.
2. Marinate chicken breasts in the mixture for 30 minutes.
3. Preheat grill to medium-high heat.
4. Grill chicken for 6-8 minutes per side or until fully cooked.

-Nutritional Value-
- Calories: 250
- Protein: 30g
- Fat: 12g
- Carbohydrates: 2g
- Cooking Time: 20 minutes

2. Quinoa and Vegetable Stir-Fry

-Ingredients-
- 1 cup quinoa (uncooked)
- 2 cups mixed vegetables (broccoli, bell peppers, carrots)
- 2 tablespoons soy sauce
- 1 tablespoon sesame oil
- 1 teaspoon ginger (minced)
- 2 cloves garlic (minced)

-Preparation-
1. Cook quinoa according to package instructions.
2. In a pan, stir-fry mixed vegetables in sesame oil.
3. Add cooked quinoa, soy sauce, ginger, and garlic. Stir until well combined.

-Nutritional Value-
- Calories: 300
- Protein: 12g
- Fat: 8g
- Carbohydrates: 45g
- Cooking Time: 25 minutes

3. Baked Salmon with Dill Sauce

-Ingredients-
- 4 salmon fillets
- 1 tablespoon olive oil
- 2 tablespoons fresh dill (chopped)
- 1 lemon (sliced)

- Salt and pepper to taste

-Preparation-
1. Preheat oven to 400°F (200°C).
2. Rub salmon with olive oil, dill, salt, and pepper.
3. Place lemon slices on top of each fillet.
4. Bake for 15-20 minutes or until salmon flakes easily with a fork.

-Nutritional Value-
- Calories: 280
- Protein: 25g
- Fat: 18g
- Carbohydrates: 2g
- Cooking Time: 20 minutes

4. Mango Avocado Salad

-Ingredients-
- 2 ripe mangoes (peeled and diced)
- 1 avocado (peeled and sliced)
- 2 cups mixed salad greens
- 1/4 cup red onion (thinly sliced)
- 2 tablespoons balsamic vinaigrette

-Preparation-
1. In a bowl, combine mangoes, avocado, salad greens, and red onion.

2. Drizzle balsamic vinaigrette over the salad and toss gently.

-Nutritional Value-
- Calories: 200
- Protein: 2g
- Fat: 10g
- Carbohydrates: 30g
- Cooking Time: 10 minutes

5. Turkey and Vegetable Skewers

-Ingredients-
- 1 pound turkey breast (cut into chunks)
- 1 zucchini (sliced)
- 1 bell pepper (cut into squares)
- 1 tablespoon olive oil
- 1 teaspoon dried rosemary
- Salt and pepper to taste

-Preparation-
1. Preheat grill or oven to medium-high heat.
2. Thread turkey, zucchini, and bell pepper onto skewers.
3. Brush with olive oil, sprinkle with rosemary, salt, and pepper.
4. Grill or bake for 15-20 minutes, turning occasionally.

-Nutritional Value-
- Calories: 220

- Protein: 30g
- Fat: 8g
- Carbohydrates: 8g
- Cooking Time: 20 minutes

6. Vegetarian Lentil Soup

-Ingredients-
- 1 cup dried lentils
- 1 onion (chopped)
- 2 carrots (diced)
- 2 celery stalks (sliced)
- 3 cloves garlic (minced)
- 6 cups vegetable broth
- 1 teaspoon cumin
- Salt and pepper to taste

-Preparation-
1. Rinse lentils and combine with vegetables, garlic, and vegetable broth in a pot.
2. Bring to a boil, then simmer for 25-30 minutes.
3. Season with cumin, salt, and pepper.

-Nutritional Value-
- Calories: 220
- Protein: 14g
- Fat: 1g
- Carbohydrates: 40g
- Cooking Time: 30 minutes

7. Spinach and Feta Stuffed Chicken

-Ingredients-
- 4 boneless, skinless chicken breasts
- 2 cups fresh spinach
- 1/2 cup feta cheese (crumbled)
- 1 tablespoon olive oil
- 1 teaspoon garlic powder
- Salt and pepper to taste

-Preparation-
1. Preheat oven to 375°F (190°C).
2. Saute spinach in olive oil until wilted.
3. Cut a pocket in each chicken breast and stuff with spinach and feta.
4. Season with garlic powder, salt, and pepper.
5. Bake for 25-30 minutes.

-Nutritional Value-
- Calories: 280
- Protein: 30g
- Fat: 12g
- Carbohydrates: 4g
- Cooking Time: 30 minutes

8. Greek Yogurt Parfait

-Ingredients-
- 1 cup Greek yogurt
- 1/2 cup granola (low-fat)

- 1/2 cup mixed berries
- 1 tablespoon honey

-Preparation-
1. In a glass or bowl, layer Greek yogurt, granola, and mixed berries.
2. Drizzle honey on top.

-Nutritional Value-
- Calories: 250
- Protein: 15g
- Fat: 8g
- Carbohydrates: 30g
- Cooking Time: 5 minutes

9. Cauliflower and Broccoli Bake

-Ingredients-
- 1 head cauliflower (cut into florets)
- 2 cups broccoli florets
- 1 cup low-fat cheddar cheese (shredded)
- 1/2 cup skim milk
- 2 tablespoons whole wheat flour
- Salt and pepper to taste

-Preparation-
1. Steam cauliflower and broccoli until tender.
2. In a saucepan, whisk together milk, flour, salt, and pepper until thickened.

3. Mix steamed vegetables with cheese sauce.
4. Bake for 20 minutes at 350°F (175°C).

-Nutritional Value-
- Calories: 180
- Protein: 12g
- Fat: 6g
- Carbohydrates: 20g
- Cooking Time: 30 minutes

10. Berry Smoothie Bowl

-Ingredients-
- 1 cup mixed berries (frozen)
- 1 banana
- 1/2 cup Greek yogurt
- 1/4 cup almond milk
- 2 tablespoons chia seeds
- 1 tablespoon honey

-Preparation-
1. Blend berries, banana, Greek yogurt, and almond milk until smooth.
2. Pour into a bowl and top with chia seeds and honey.

-Nutritional Value-
- Calories: 230
- Protein: 10g
- Fat: 8g

- Carbohydrates: 35g
- Preparation Time: 5 minutes

These recipes are crafted to meet the dietary needs of seniors without a gallbladder, focusing on nutrient density, balanced ingredients, and ease of digestion. Adjust portion sizes based on individual preferences and nutritional requirements. Enjoy a variety of flavorful and nourishing meals with these recipes from the "No Gallbladder Cookbook for Seniors."

DINNER

1. Herb-Roasted Chicken with Sweet Potatoes

-Ingredients-
- 4 bone-in, skinless chicken thighs
- 2 sweet potatoes (peeled and cubed)
- 2 tablespoons olive oil
- 1 teaspoon dried rosemary
- 1 teaspoon dried thyme
- Salt and pepper to taste

-Preparation-
1. Preheat oven to 400°F (200°C).
2. Toss sweet potatoes with olive oil, rosemary, thyme, salt, and pepper.
3. Place chicken thighs on top of sweet potatoes.
4. Roast for 35-40 minutes or until chicken reaches an internal temperature of 165°F (74°C).

-Nutritional Value-
- Calories: 350
- Protein: 25g
- Fat: 15g
- Carbohydrates: 25g
- Cooking Time: 40 minutes

2. Salmon and Asparagus Foil Packets

-Ingredients-
- 4 salmon fillets
- 1 bunch asparagus (trimmed)
- 2 tablespoons lemon juice
- 2 tablespoons olive oil
- 1 teaspoon dill
- Salt and pepper to taste

-Preparation-
1. Preheat oven to 375°F (190°C).
2. Place each salmon fillet on a piece of foil, surround with asparagus.
3. Drizzle with lemon juice and olive oil, sprinkle with dill, salt, and pepper.
4. Seal packets and bake for 20-25 minutes.

-Nutritional Value-
- Calories: 280
- Protein: 30g
- Fat: 16g
- Carbohydrates: 8g
- Cooking Time: 25 minutes

3. Vegetarian Quinoa Stuffed Peppers

-Ingredients-
- 4 bell peppers (halved and seeds removed)
- 1 cup quinoa (cooked)

- 1 can black beans (rinsed and drained)
- 1 cup corn kernels
- 1 cup diced tomatoes
- 1 teaspoon cumin
- Salt and pepper to taste

-Preparation-
1. Preheat oven to 375°F (190°C).
2. In a bowl, mix quinoa, black beans, corn, tomatoes, cumin, salt, and pepper.
3. Stuff peppers with the quinoa mixture.
4. Bake for 25-30 minutes.

-Nutritional Value-
- Calories: 320
- Protein: 15g
- Fat: 2g
- Carbohydrates: 65g
- Cooking Time: 30 minutes

4. Chicken and Vegetable Stir-Fry

-Ingredients-
- 1 pound boneless, skinless chicken breast (sliced)
- 2 cups broccoli florets
- 1 red bell pepper (sliced)
- 1 cup snap peas
- 3 tablespoons low-sodium soy sauce
- 1 tablespoon sesame oil

- 1 teaspoon ginger (minced)

-Preparation-
1. In a wok or skillet, stir-fry chicken until cooked.
2. Add vegetables and continue to stir-fry until tender.
3. Drizzle with soy sauce, sesame oil, and ginger.
4. Cook for an additional 2-3 minutes.

-Nutritional Value-
- Calories: 320
- Protein: 30g
- Fat: 10g
- Carbohydrates: 25g
- Cooking Time: 20 minutes

5. Turkey and Vegetable Meatball Soup

-Ingredients-
- 1 pound ground turkey
- 1/2 cup breadcrumbs
- 1 egg
- 1 onion (diced)
- 2 carrots (sliced)
- 2 celery stalks (sliced)
- 6 cups low-sodium chicken broth
- 1 teaspoon dried thyme
- Salt and pepper to taste

-Preparation-
1. In a bowl, mix ground turkey, breadcrumbs, and egg. Form into meatballs.
2. In a pot, sauté onions, carrots, and celery until softened.
3. Add chicken broth, meatballs, thyme, salt, and pepper.
4. Simmer for 20-25 minutes.

-Nutritional Value-
- Calories: 280
- Protein: 25g
- Fat: 12g
- Carbohydrates: 15g
- Cooking Time: 25 minutes

6. Mushroom and Spinach Omelette

-Ingredients-
- 4 large eggs
- 1 cup mushrooms (sliced)
- 1 cup fresh spinach
- 1/4 cup feta cheese (crumbled)
- 1 tablespoon olive oil
- Salt and pepper to taste

-Preparation-
1. In a skillet, sauté mushrooms and spinach in olive oil until wilted.
2. Whisk eggs and pour over the vegetables.
3. Cook until edges set, then sprinkle with feta.

4. Fold the omelette and cook for an additional 2 minutes.

-Nutritional Value-
- Calories: 280
- Protein: 18g
- Fat: 20g
- Carbohydrates: 6g
- Cooking Time: 10 minutes

7. Lemon Garlic Shrimp with Zucchini Noodles

-Ingredients-
- 1 pound shrimp (peeled and deveined)
- 4 medium zucchini (spiralized)
- 2 tablespoons olive oil
- 2 cloves garlic (minced)
- 1 lemon (juiced)
- 1 teaspoon dried parsley
- Salt and pepper to taste

-Preparation-
1. In a skillet, sauté shrimp in olive oil and garlic until pink.
2. Add zucchini noodles, lemon juice, parsley, salt, and pepper.
3. Cook for 3-5 minutes until zucchini is tender.

-Nutritional Value-
- Calories: 250

- Protein: 30g
- Fat: 12g
- Carbohydrates: 10g
- Cooking Time: 15 minutes

8. Chickpea and Vegetable Curry

-Ingredients-
- 1 can chickpeas (rinsed and drained)
- 1 eggplant (cubed)
- 1 bell pepper (sliced)
- 1 onion (diced)
- 1 can coconut milk
- 2 tablespoons curry powder
- Salt and pepper to taste

-Preparation-
1. In a pot, sauté eggplant, bell pepper, and onion until softened.
2. Add chickpeas, coconut milk, curry powder, salt, and pepper.
3. Simmer for 20-25 minutes.

-Nutritional Value-
- Calories: 300
- Protein: 10g
- Fat: 18g
- Carbohydrates: 30g
- Cooking Time: 25 minutes

9. Baked Cod with Tomato and Olive Relish

-Ingredients-
- 4 cod fillets
- 1 cup cherry tomatoes (halved)
- 1/2 cup Kalamata olives (pitted and sliced)
- 2 tablespoons olive oil
- 1 tablespoon balsamic vinegar
- 1 teaspoon dried basil
- Salt and pepper to taste

-Preparation-
1. Preheat oven to 375°F (190°C).
2. Season cod with salt and pepper, bake for 15-20 minutes.
3. In a bowl, mix tomatoes, olives, olive oil, balsamic vinegar, and basil.
4. Spoon the relish over baked cod.

-Nutritional Value-
- Calories: 280
- Protein: 30g
- Fat: 15g
- Carbohydrates: 10g
- Cooking Time: 20 minutes

10. Veggie-Packed Brown Rice Bowl

-Ingredients-
- 2 cups cooked brown rice
- 1 cup broccoli florets

- 1 cup shredded carrots
- 1 cup snow peas
- 1 cup tofu (cubed)
- 2 tablespoons soy sauce
- 1 tablespoon sesame oil

-Preparation-
1. In a pan, sauté tofu until golden brown.
2. Add broccoli, carrots, and snow peas. Stir-fry until vegetables are tender.
3. Mix in cooked brown rice, soy sauce, and sesame oil.
4. Cook for an additional 5 minutes.

-Nutritional Value-
- Calories: 320
- Protein: 15g
- Fat: 12g
- Carbohydrates: 40g
- Cooking Time: 15 minutes

These dinner recipes are designed for seniors without a gallbladder, featuring balanced ingredients, easy preparation, and nutritious choices to support digestive health. Adjust portion sizes based on individual needs and enjoy flavorful, satisfying dinners with these recipes.

SNACK

1. Greek Yogurt and Berry Parfait

-Ingredients-
- 1 cup Greek yogurt
- 1/2 cup mixed berries (strawberries, blueberries, raspberries)
- 2 tablespoons granola (low-fat)
- 1 tablespoon honey

-Preparation-
1. In a glass or bowl, layer Greek yogurt, mixed berries, and granola.
2. Drizzle honey on top.

-Nutritional Value-
- Calories: 200
- Protein: 12g
- Fat: 6g
- Carbohydrates: 30g
- Preparation Time: 5 minutes

2. Cucumber and Hummus Bites

-Ingredients-
- 1 cucumber (sliced)
- 1/2 cup hummus (store-bought or homemade)
- Cherry tomatoes for garnish

-Preparation-
1. Spread a small amount of hummus on each cucumber slice.
2. Top with a cherry tomato for added freshness.

-Nutritional Value-
- Calories: 120
- Protein: 5g
- Fat: 8g
- Carbohydrates: 10g
- Preparation Time: 10 minutes

3. Oat and Nut Energy Balls

-Ingredients-
- 1 cup rolled oats
- 1/2 cup nut butter (almond or peanut)
- 1/4 cup honey
- 1/2 cup chopped nuts (walnuts, almonds)
- 1/4 cup dark chocolate chips (optional)

-Preparation-
1. In a bowl, mix rolled oats, nut butter, honey, chopped nuts, and chocolate chips.
2. Form into small balls and refrigerate for 30 minutes.

-Nutritional Value-
- Calories: 150

- Protein: 6g
- Fat: 10g
- Carbohydrates: 12g
- Preparation Time: 15 minutes

4. Vegetable Sticks with Avocado Dip

-Ingredients-
- 2 carrots (cut into sticks)
- 2 celery stalks (cut into sticks)
- 1 bell pepper (sliced)
- 1 ripe avocado
- 1 tablespoon lime juice
- Salt and pepper to taste

-Preparation-
1. Arrange carrot sticks, celery sticks, and bell pepper slices on a plate.
2. In a bowl, mash avocado and mix with lime juice, salt, and pepper.
3. Use the avocado dip as a tasty accompaniment.

-Nutritional Value-
- Calories: 180
- Protein: 4g
- Fat: 12g
- Carbohydrates: 18g
- Preparation Time: 10 minutes

5. Chia Seed Pudding with Mango

-Ingredients-
- 2 tablespoons chia seeds
- 1/2 cup almond milk
- 1/2 teaspoon vanilla extract
- 1 tablespoon honey
- 1/2 cup diced mango

-Preparation-
1. In a jar, mix chia seeds, almond milk, vanilla extract, and honey.
2. Refrigerate for at least 2 hours or overnight.
3. Top with diced mango before serving.

-Nutritional Value-
- Calories: 180
- Protein: 4g
- Fat: 8g
- Carbohydrates: 25g
- Preparation Time: 2 hours (includes chilling time)

These snack recipes are tailored for seniors without a gallbladder, focusing on nutrient-dense ingredients and easy preparation. Adjust portion sizes based on individual preferences and dietary needs. Enjoy these wholesome and delicious snacks that contribute to digestive well-being.

Conclusion

The "No Gallbladder Cookbook for Seniors" provides a thoughtful and practical approach to supporting digestive health and overall well-being for individuals navigating life without a gallbladder. The recipes outlined in this cookbook are carefully crafted to address the specific dietary needs of seniors, emphasizing nutrient-dense, easily digestible, and flavorful options.

By incorporating lean proteins, low-fat dairy, a variety of fruits and vegetables, and mindful sources of healthy fats, this cookbook strives to alleviate potential digestive discomfort while ensuring seniors receive the essential nutrients vital for their overall health. The inclusion of herbs, spices, and specific cooking methods further enhances the culinary experience, offering both nourishment and enjoyment in each meal.

Moreover, the balanced nutrition provided by the cookbook not only supports digestive comfort but also addresses broader aspects of well-being, including heart health, weight management, and stable blood sugar levels. The recipes are designed to be approachable and adaptable, encouraging seniors to explore a diverse range of flavors and textures while maintaining a diet that aligns with their unique dietary requirements.

As a special motivation, embracing the "No Gallbladder Cookbook for Seniors" is an empowering step towards prioritizing one's health and savoring the joys of food without compromising digestive ease. By adopting and adapting to this diet, seniors can experience the positive impact of nourishing their bodies with meals crafted with care and consideration. The cookbook serves not only as a guide to practical recipes but also as a companion in the journey toward embracing a diet that fosters well-being, resilience, and a fulfilling culinary experience. May the joy of preparing and enjoying these meals inspire a renewed sense of vitality, encouraging seniors to savor each bite on the path to sustained digestive wellness.

* 9 7 9 8 8 7 8 4 1 4 3 7 1 *